THE TOYBAG GUIDE TO

MEDICAL PLAY

BY TEMPEST

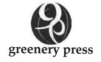

greenery press

CONTENTS

FOREWORD

When I joined my local BDSM community, I was pleasantly surprised at the number of health care professionals represented in our ranks. But not that many of them wanted to do medical play, because it was too much like what they did at work. So when I began writing this guide, I was one of very few locally who delved into medical play. By the time I finished, though, I had corrupted and converted and uncovered enough medical players to start a trend.

As more and more people get tired of the standard tie 'em up and flog 'em, I suspect that medical play will be incorporated into their scenes to spice things up a bit. And then when the medical fetish bug bites, and they find there is no cure, medical play will be as common as over-the-knee spanking. At least, that is my prognosis!

Thank you to Janet Hardy of Greenery Press for giving me this opportunity to share what I have learned about medical play. Thank you to my switchy husband, John, for putting up with my long hours at the computer while I researched and wrote, and the rest of my wonderful leather family, especially my submissive, Lou.

— *Tempest, a kinky health care professional since 1984*

Chapter 1. The Medical Fetish

America has a medical fetish, as witnessed by the resounding acclaim for medical dramas such as *ER*, *St. Elsewhere*, even *M*A*S*H**. The blood and gore, the technical jargon, the professionals in their starched white uniforms and cool, comfy scrubs give us goosebumps and have held our attention for years. Some of us, however, get more than just a mild thrill from the flair of a nurse's cap and the surgeon's skilled handling of a scalpel.

It is a rare individual who doesn't have pleasant memories of "playing doctor" with a neighborhood friend as a child, examining that mysterious and exciting taboo of the human body, especially the genitals. Why did we play doctor anyway? Maybe we were too shy and the thrill too much to endure to explore each other's bodies without the pretense of a medical exam. The safe and familiar confines of the doctor's office gave us the courage to drop our drawers and be initiated into the age old sexual fetish of medical play.

Now, as adults, we use the medical knowledge we've gleaned from TV, books, and of course, the Internet, to "play doctor" and continue that favorite childhood exploration of human sexuality. Judging from the popularity of Internet community email lists and medical porn sites, we get quite a charge from naughty nurses, Good

Doctor/Evil Doctor, and patients who turn the tables on their health care professional.

Americans aren't the only one with a yen for medical play. A quick search of the World Wide Web finds worldwide fascination for the same tricks of the trade, only with a European or Asian flair. *Iryou fetchi* (medical fetish) is big in Japan. In a Japanese goth nightclub you might see "nurses" who look like they've been practicing surgery on themselves, patients who think being broken is cute, plenty of fake blood and gauze bandages, and dolls or stuffed animals that have suffered grievous bodily harm.

This is not a new phenomenon, either. We just know more about it and have better access to medical toys for our play. In the movie *The Road to Wellville*, Anthony Hopkins plays the infamous true-life Dr. Kellogg, who ran a health spa at the turn of the century in Battle Creek, Michigan. His spa catered to affluent people coming for "the cure," which included numerous enemas and torturous treatment with the many machines that the good doctor had invented. Featured in the movie was the treatment for "hysteria," which included vaginal fisting. Ah, those were the days.

In this book I will attempt to pass along the information I've learned, from both BDSM and medical sources, about medical play. One may wonder, "What does BDSM have to do with playing doctor?" Well, the answer is, "A lot." In BDSM (Bondage/Discipline/Sadism/

Masochism), there is a top (a giver of sensations) and a bottom (the receiver of sensations). Alternatively there may be a dominant (controller of the situation) and a submissive (one who is not in control of the situation). In medical play there is at least one person who is giving sensations (the exam, the treatment, the pain, the pleasure) and in control of the situation, and at least one person who has consented to receive the ministrations of that person.

Consent is an important part of any BDSM play, especially medical play. Informed consent is best, so the bottom should "bone up" on the subject before subjecting his "boner" to the talents of another: one cannot consent to something that one doesn't understand. Nor should a top consent to perform an act upon another unless that top thoroughly understands how to do so. Especially with medical play, an untrained top can unknowingly inflict permanent damage on the bottom.

Part of playing safely is full disclosure of health issues, including: past injuries, current conditions, diseases that may be passed though body fluids, current medications, mental/emotional status, past positive or negative experiences with medical play. Be upfront about your limits as either a top or bottom. Tops have limits, too, and should not be pressured to exceed them by a pushy bottom. All bottoms have limits. If you don't believe that, get out the bone saw and proceed to cut off their limbs. You will find very quickly that the bottom does indeed have limits.

Disclaimer:

I am not a physician, nor do I play one on TV. However, I do play one in the dungeon. It is only play, as my medical training is not in diagnosis or treatment. I am not representing myself here as a medical doctor, therapist or clinician of any kind. I am not here to ease your pain, boys and girls! For help with genuine medical problems, please consult your physician. Let's get started… just bend over, open wide and say, "ahhhhhhh."

Chapter 2. Setting the Mood with the Exam Room

You can incorporate individual aspects of medical play into your play repertoire without too much trouble, using your usual equipment and playroom set up. Or you can go the distance to create an unforgettable medical scene with your own faux exam room.

Set the mood by setting up a mock medical office with a few items to suggest a clinical environment. Hanging white sheets separate the medical play area from the rest of the house and separate the bottom from their every-day worries. Have the bottom step into another world by using your imagination and a few select items of medical décor.

While a medical table or exam table is always the *piéce de resistance*, these large items of furniture are hard to explain to the in-laws and cost a pretty penny. If you want to invest in a medical table, however, contact hospitals about their surplus equipment. Doctor's offices and clinics sell their used equipment to the public at reduced prices. It never hurts to ask. On-line auction services, such as eBay, are another source, but expect high shipping charges. If a

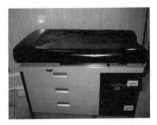

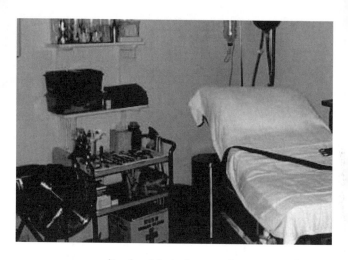

true medical table is beyond your reach, consider purchasing a fold-up massage table. For less than $200 you can set up your kinky clinic anywhere you have space.

Any table, as long as it is sturdy, makes an excellent exam table. To convert a regular dining room table, coffee table, or desk to an exam table, pad the surface with a blanket and cover with more disposable absorbent padding. This padding has an absorbent side and a plastic coated side. Put the plastic side down and the absorbent side against the bottom's bottom. Why pad the table? Most bottoms like to be comfortable while they are being tortured! You may need a small pillow and a folded towel to place under the small of the bottom's back. I find that the more comfortable the bottom is during a scene, the less they have to worry about extraneous pain, and the more they can concentrate on the deliciously evil things I am doing to them.

The most comfortable exam table is your bed, of course. If you can provide water-resistant vinyl sheeting and pillow covers that crinkle with every movement, all the better. Cover the vinyl with starched white sheets and then the disposable absorbent padding. Many beds have attachment points built in, and tell the truth, didn't you consider that when you bought the bed? But if you are unlucky enough to have no place which to attach a rope, then bring two long pieces of rope under the bed, with the ends extending out on each side. Each end can attach to a limb for bondage.

You'll need something on which to place your medical tools. A stainless steel tray or a tray stand is perfect for the medical mind-fuck. Can't afford a doctor's stainless steel tray? Get a brand new shiny baking sheet and keep it for just this purpose. Or cover

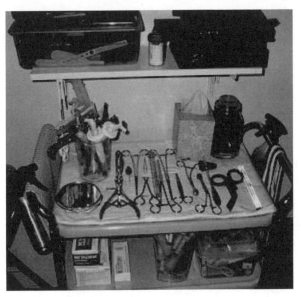

a used baking sheet with towels or the
disposable drapes... then who can tell
the difference?

You can't have too much stainless
steel in the medical room. Besides the
tray stand, there are stainless steel canister containers, trash cans, gooseneck
lamps, scales, and short stools on which

an evil doc can sit during an exam. An alternative to the stainless steel trash can is a regular trash can stenciled with a biohazard symbol and the words "medical waste."

An IV stand can be purchased from a medical supply store or on-line kink store. It makes a great piece of equipment to hold not only bags of sterile IV solution, but also enema bags, floggers, and other implements.

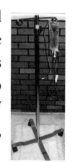

Walls can not only be deco-

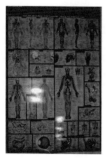

rated with white sheets, but also operating room green sheets and medical charts, such as the eye chart and anatomy charts that we have all seen in the doctor's office.

The mind-fuck starts when you have your patient strip and dress him/her in either a cloth or paper patient gown that is open in the back. They may lose the gown during the exam, but donning the gown at the beginning is a great way to start the scene. Like wearing a collar, wearing the exam gown can put the bottom into the correct frame of mind for a medical scene.

If the patient is going to be dressed properly, well, so should the top. Starched white uniforms are still the dress code of the day, but are rapidly being replaced with cool, comfy surgical scrubs. Scrubs are available everywhere these days, as they have escaped from the OR and have invaded local malls in mid-America. By themselves or covered with a white lab coat, scrubs are easy to work in or play in. Uniforms, lab coats, scrubs, and matching shoes are available at uniform or nurse's shops nationwide. If you prefer something a bit more risqué, look for the uniform of the naughty nurse in costume shops and on-line. You'll find the naughty nurse wearing satin and latex in addition to the traditional fabrics. Drape a stethoscope around your neck, and you are set to begin. Stethoscopes can be costly or inexpensive depending upon the type purchased. Since you aren't trying to pick up heart murmurs, go for the cheaper models (less than $20).

Chapter 3. Tools of the Trade

In later chapters I'll discuss specific nasty pieces of equipment and the techniques needed to use them, but you may also want to stock up on some general tools of the trade, so to speak.

Alcohol and alcohol wipes are key to a medical scene. Smell is ultra-important in triggering memories and emotions, and bringing an alcohol wipe under the nose of a blindfolded or bound bottom can trigger memories of past medical experiences and trips to the doctor or hospital. Antiseptics such as iodine and disinfectant spray can also elicit a strong response from the bottom and put them into the proper frame of mind.

Bandages will be needed during many scenes, after a needlestick or cutting, or just as part of the mind-fuck. One of my favorite scenes is to pretend that I accidentally cut the patient, fuss over the faux laceration, and bandage it up. All the while the bottom is trying to decide whether I am serious or just messing with his mind. Either way, I succeeded.

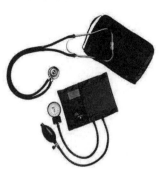

One of the first actions that a nurse takes in a doctor's office is to take your blood pressure. Inexpensive blood pressure cuffs can be purchased from your local pharmacy. Besides taking a real (but elevated by the scene) blood pressure, the cuff can be used as a part of bondage. When that cuff is inflated on a body part, that part pretty much remains immobile. A pediatric blood pressure cuff can be place on a cock — then, pump him up!

Cotton balls in a glass canister or container not only help the décor of the exam room, but come in handy for waving alcohol under the nose of the bottom, applying 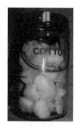 antiseptics to a real or faux break in the skin, and even can be used in the procedure for fire cupping.

A friend of mine is a kinky dental hygienist and keeps me stocked in evil dental tools. She was the one who introduced me to the vibrating flosser which has become a mainstay in my genitorture play. Dental hygienists must be some of the most sadistic people I know, using hooks and other sharp tools to s-c-r-a-p-e the plaque and tartar from our teeth. These tools can also be used to scare the dickens out of a bottom, and with which to do sensation play all over the body. Can't picture it? OK, how about using the very end of a hygienist's hook to tickle the clit? "Now hold very, very still… I wouldn't want to hurt you with this thing!" Dental floss is the smallest kind of twine you can use in a scene for fine tying: cock and balls, lacing a needle corset, or simply tying nipples. Be careful with floss: because it is fine, it can get tight and hard to remove.

24

Whether you are doing ass play, a medical scene, or simply humiliation, keep a few disposable enemas on hand for when the need arises. Cheap, generic, pre-lubricated 150ml enemas will work for most scenes. But when the scene itself revolves around enemas, you may want to invest in an enema kit. These kits can range from under $10 and include vaginal/rectal

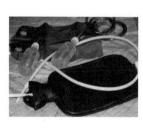 tube to the Gold Standard of enema kits that have adaptors that can add up to big bucks. If enemas are your kink, the money is well spent. See the chapter on Weapons of Ass Destruction.

A face mask is really part of your apparel, but I am including it here

because you won't wear it all of the time. There are the surgical type masks that are folded paper 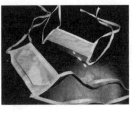 with strings attached for tying behind your head. There are also the firmer, molded masks that are held in place with a rubber band. Masks are frequently found in the BDSM lifestyle, so surgical masks fit right in.

Forceps are fancy tweezers, and hemostats look like scissors that clamp instead of cut. It doesn't take too much imagination to see the useful- 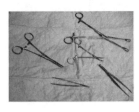 ness of these tools in medical play. But be careful with hemostats and be sure to try them out on yourself before using them on another person. Start with the lowest setting and work your way up higher. Stainless steel hemostats can be quite harsh. Look for the blue plastic disposable type of hemostats for regular use. Reserve the steel ones for serious pain sluts.

Disposable gloves are a necessity for cleanliness, preventing the spread of disease, and the mind-fuck. Latex gloves are the least expensive and are available in a variety of colors, including bitchin' black. But not everyone can use latex products. Due to the abundance of latex in everything from balloons to rubber bands to condoms, latex allergies are a serious concern to those doing real or play medical exams. Find out during your negotiations if the bottom is allergic to latex or anything else. Alternatives to latex gloves are nitrile or vinyl gloves, which are somewhat thicker and not as sensitive, but perform the job nicely. Disposable gloves come in the long version as well, especially nice for fisting.

Lubricants ease the way to many a great scene, but one type does not fit all scenes. Know your lubes and have the correct one on hand. Petroleum-based lubes, like petroleum jelly (Vaseline®), baby oil, or mineral oil are used often for sex and play, but doctors never use them — so if you want total authenticity, stick to the water-based lubes I'll describe soon. As petroleum-based lubes destroy latex practically on contact, they should never be used with condoms, diaphragms or cervical caps. They also stain fabric and can be difficult to wash out.

Oil-based lubricants, usually made from natural products, such as vegetable oils, nut oils, Crisco® and butter, also tend to stain fabrics and can be difficult to wash off, but they are safe for use with the vagina. Like petroleum-based lubes, they are a no-no with latex. Oil-based lubricants are great for anal sex, vaginal intercourse, and male and female masturbation in those cases where you don't need latex.

Water-based lubricants, such as Astroglide® or KY®, are what you'll find in your doctor's office. They typically contain deionized water, glycerin, propylene glycol and nontoxic preservatives. Although available in both flavored and unflavored mixtures, most unflavored lubes still taste slightly sweet. Water-based lubes do not stain, are safe for use with latex and all other barrier birth control methods, and rarely cause irritation in any body orifice. The only problem with these lubes is their staying power, as they may dry out during an extended sex session.

Silicone-based lubricants, such as Eros®, are similar to water-based lubes, with one big difference: they are completely waterproof, making them ideal for underwater use. They also retain their lubricating properties better and longer, and are highly concentrated... so a little goes a long way! Silicone will not harm latex as oil and petroleum-based lubricants do; however, silicone-based lubricants can harm sex toys made from silicone, so use a different lube when using your toys or cover your toy with a condom.

Even if you have no intention of doing a temporary piercing, needles can come in handy for a medical scene. When the bottom enters the room and sees the needles laid out with all of the other evil implements, his/her heart will go pitter-pat. Hold up some sterile needles or sterile lancets, in front of a bottom's face and make them think that they are in for some piercing! You can always drag the point against the skin or prick the skin in strategic spots. Just pricking the skin is a good build up to an actual temporary piercing for a squeamish bottom. Don't forget the alcohol first. Needles without a syringe attached can be purchased without a prescription in many states. In other states you must sign a form to buy them or have a prescription. You can avoid the hassle and potential embarrassment by simply ordering them online from a kinky medical site. Lancets, which are used in the vanilla world to prick the skin to retrieve a drop of blood for diabetic testing, are the less evil and easier-to-handle little brother of needles. Lancets are easily obtained from your local pharmacy.

Who doesn't have a neurological (Wartenburg) wheel in their toy bag? If you are already using a wheel in your play, then, congratulations, you are already incorporating medical play into your regular play. This little wheel with sharp spikes is on the end of a heavy stainless steel handle. The weight of the handle is enough to put pressure on the business end while you are running it over the skin of the bottom. So, do not press down, but simply hold the end of the handle, letting the weight of the instrument provide the pressure. A Wartenburg wheel can break the skin if you are not careful or if the bottom has particularly thin skin in areas. For this reason, you should make an informed decision about the safety of this sort of play. For maximum safety, keep one wheel per bottom; or, as a slightly less safe alternative, sanitize the wheel before or after play according to the instructions starting on page 63. Less expensive disposable plastic neurological wheels are also available from kinky medical sites online.

An Oxygen Breather Mask with bag, for show or for breath play, is sure to make your bottom gasp. A long tube connects to the top of the mask and the other end can be connected to an air source. As one breathes into the bag, it contracts and expands with each breath. You can easily modify the mask to increase the amount of air flow allowed because, strangely enough, the bottoms tend to get excited and breathe more heavily in these types of scenes. Check the Resource Guide and do your homework before attempting breath-play — it's riskier than a lot of people realize.

Got rope? Then you need bandage scissors, also called medical shears, or EMT scissors. These scissors are bent in such a way as to allow them to run along the skin to easily cut off bandages, rope, plastic wrap, clothing or whatever is coming between you and the bottom's skin. The lower tip is blunted to avoid cutting the skin. These inexpensive scissors should be in everyone's toy bag, whether you do medical play or not. The heavy stainless steel version looks awesome lying out on your implement tray.

A small, red biohazard container, also known as a "sharps" container, comes in handy for disposing for needles, lancets and anything with which blood has come into contact. The last thing you want to do is throw a used needle or lancet into a plastic trash bag, only to be stabbed with a contaminated "sharp" when you take out the trash (or to put your garbage

collector at nonconsensual risk!).
While sharps containers are cheap and
easily obtained from a pharmacy, in a
pinch you can use a soda bottle with
a screw-on cap. Many local hospitals
collect sharps containers for incin-
eration with their regular biohazard
waste. Alternatively, glue the lid onto
a full sharps container and dispose of
it in your regular trash.

Before many medical procedures,
all the hair in a certain area must be
removed for sanitary reasons. Hair can
hold germs! So shaving supplies can be
part of your medical toy box. As part
of the play, the top can shave the bottom's bottom, pubic hair, chest or back
hair. Opening oneself up to a razor in
the hand of the top is a very submissive action, and one that calls for a

great deal of trust. Being shaved is also humiliating, which appeals to a large percentage of the BDSM community. The ultimate in shaving humiliation is having one's head shaved, but the ass — especially the perineal area — runs a close second. Many tops want their male bottoms completely shaved in the nether regions including right up to the anus or opening of the rectum. To shave the scrotum, pull down firmly to make the skin taut and avoid nicks.

A stethoscope is more than a piece of sexy medical apparel or costume. You can use it to listen to the heart rate go up and down during a scene. One imaginative trick is to put the earpieces in the ears of the bottom and tape the diaphragm to his/her chest. This forces them to listen to their own heartbeat throbbing and pounding in their ears as the scene continues. Please make sure that you have comfortable earpieces (try them on yourself for five minutes or more), or the bottom will be more concerned with the bad pain their ears than the good pain you are giving them.

Syringes, without a needle, can be devious little implements. Pick up an oral syringe from the pharmacy, the kind that you use to give medicine to kids. Remove the plunger first. Using a small hacksaw, cut the bottom off of the syringe, then file down any sharp points. Put the plunger back in, but this time into the opening you just created. Place the other opening on a nipple and pull back on the plunger. Instant vacuum!

As far as thermometers go, I just want to mention two words: rectal temperature! If you think that the bottom is really hot stuff, try using a candy thermometer to measure rectal temperature. Where else can you take a temperature? You might want to start in the mouth, then under the arm, then between the legs, then rectal. There are two more places to try. What is the bottom's vaginal temperature or penile temperature? Before attempting a measurement of penile temperature, please read the information on sounding in the chapter on urethral play.

Tongue depressors, known in the arts and crafts store as craft sticks and by the rest of the world as popsicle sticks, are used by doctors to sadistically hold down the tongue, practically gagging the patient, to give a better glimpse down the throat. I know that members of our community can do a better job of it than the doctors. Tongue depressors can also be inserted into other body orifices, and have just enough give to them to be snapped against the patient's skin, again and again and again...

See the Resources List at the end of the book for a list of medical suppliers of everything in this book.

Chapter 4. Role-Play

While much of "what it is that we do" (WIITWD) can easily be utilized in role play, medical play presents the best chance to play a role with which we have been familiar with since birth: the Good Doctor or the Scary Doctor or that of the helpless, oh-so-compliant patient.

The Good Doctor/Bad Doctor role allows the top to be nice and gentle to the bottom while at the same time performing intimate, humiliating, and possibly painful procedures such as a general examination or triage of the patient's condition. A thorough exam of the patient will cover every orifice, the mammary glands, and the patient's reflexes and responses to various stimuli. Most tops in the scene can dream up multiple devious stimuli with which to test the bottom's responses. The Good Doctor/Bad Doctor gives, not only general exams, but specific exams such the gyne exam and the proctology exam.

The doctor spends a good deal of time on the golf course, leaving the patient in the capable hands of the nurse. Naughty Nurse emulates the Good Doctor, treating her patients with tender loving care, while administering rectal enemas and probing the depths of a cock with urethral sounds. But look out for The Nurse From Hell! You've seen her time and time again in the movies and on TV: Nurse Ratched and Bertha Ballbreaker all wrapped up in a white uniform and carrying a tray of needles with your name on them! The Nurse From Hell means business and she isn't here to coddle you, no sir. She is going to cause you some pain, and guess what? She enjoys her job. Role-play is what you make it, so there are no rules against combining The Naughty Nurse with The Nurse From Hell to create a medical scene that would win an Oscar.

Medical scenes don't necessarily have to be contemporary — remember, it's your role play. Travel back to medieval times to practice fire cupping to remove the "demons, bad essence, blocked energy flow" from your patient.

If cupping isn't your style, then place your patient in the hands of a wise but deviant sorcerer who uses acupuncture needles to cure his patients.

Dr. Frankenstein, the mad and brilliant scientist, loved his electrical play. Using the violet wand, TENS unit and vibrators, set the scene to "recreate" his experiments and bring your subject to life... again... and again.

Dare I mention a common fantasy in the vanilla community that could have much more exciting results in the BDSM world... that of turning the tables on the doctor or nurse? The unsuspecting medical professional is only trying to do his or her job, when the patient takes charge of the situation. Roles are reversed and now the patient becomes the dominant of the scene, trying out various instruments on the nurse or doctor. "Let's see how you like this medicine now!"

Chapter 5. For Your Own Good

Specific exams that patients should have for their own good are the gynecological exam for the female patient and the briefer but just as important scrotal exam for the male patient. Few women enjoy being back in the stirrups, anticipating the touch of that cold, metal speculum. Play on that anticipation; build on the humiliation of having to spread one's legs for the doctor, exposing one's most private parts. Keeping the speculum in the refrigerator is completely up to you... and whether your neighbors can hear her howl.

Both patients need proctology/rectal exams to make sure that everything is coming out OK. For male patients, this can be expanded to include the prostate exam. The prostate gland can be felt by pressing a finger into the middle of the perineum, between the scrotum and the anus. But a more reliable and fun way to check the prostate is rectally. Just insert a gloved, lubed finger or two into the rectum, and slide it back, pressing toward the front of the body. You'll feel a small lump, hopefully hard and not soft or mushy. Rhythmic massage of the prostate by the top can "milk" the bottom and deny orgasmic response.

A thorough breast exam is a must for every female visiting her kinky doctor. Each breast should be carefully examined visually, rolled in the hands, smoothed out, pinched in places (Yes, pinched! Why? For your own good!), then the nipples examined. Each nipple should be rubbed until erect, pulled to test elasticity, clamped if necessary, and even tasted. Some tests may include finding out much weight each nipple can hold, attached to clamps or nipple rings.

Some ideas:

> Bottom is going away to college, and needs to have a physical exam before she goes. She has not had a complete exam in many years, so the doctor must be thorough to check her entire body. She has all of her vitals checked, including a complete gynecology exam. He even lubricates his fingers and checks her ass. Good doctor!

Bottom is getting ready to start cheerleading for her college football team, and must undergo a very thorough medical exam before she can be on the squad. She visits her doctor who gives her a very complete medical exam. She gets all of her vitals checked as well as her breasts, vaginal exam and rectal checkup. After all, she needs to be in top shape to be on the squad.

Bottom visits his doctor because he was having some lower back pain. When the nurse comes into the room she has him strip down and she gives him a quick exam. She then calls in the female doctor who gives him a very thorough exam. She checks his prostate by sticking a finger deep into his ass. She finishes the exam by checking his temperature rectally. There she finds the trouble... his ass is not hot enough and she warms it up with a paddle. Problem solved.

Bottom visited his doctor to get his yearly checkup. Although he was embarrassed to admit it to the doctor, he was recently having a lot of anal sex with his boyfriend and wanted his doctor to make sure everything was OK. The doctor gives him a complete examination check-ing all of his vitals signs, his vital organs, his cock, his balls and finally makes his way to a through and intense rectal exam requiring an elbow length exam glove.

If our bottom is not a patient at all, but has been extremely naughty, say for example, has been arrested for some nefarious crime, and then what is called for is a body cavity search. Good Doctor is gone, and Prison Doctor snaps on those gloves. Lube is optional because you are my bitch now!

For example:

Bottom was caught trying to smuggle drugs onto an airplane in a foreign country. She is taken by security to the holding cell. A doctor then enters the room and orders her to strip down. She refuses, so the guard and doctor force her to remove her clothing. They then give her a humiliating body cavity search. They check her orally, vaginally and rectally while she is handcuffed and helpless.

Chapter 6. Weapons of Ass Destruction

Where are the weapons of ass destruction? Well, they are right in my toy bag, not counting the ones in the bathroom closet! Oh, I am not referring to the everyday ass toys with exotic names such as the Midnight

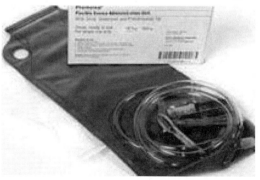

Rider or Blue Thunder Ass Master. No, I mean those nasty stainless steel devices that have made patients cringe for decades such as the anal speculum, analscope, probes and my personal favorite ass weapon... the ever-so-useful cleansing enema prior to the full body cavity search.

A simple cleansing enema prior to ass play, or just to up the humiliation factor, can be done simply with an inexpensive commercially available enema, such as Fleets® or a generic brand. Anyone can give an enema. You can even make the bottom give it to themself! First warm the disposable plastic enema bottle under warm water for a few minutes. Position the patient in the knee-chest position on their side. Insert the pre-lubricated rectal nozzle into the rectum two to three inches at an angle that points toward the bellybutton. Slowly apply gentle steady pressure on to the solution container until all the contents have been instilled into the rectum. Don't just squeeze like heck. Make sure that the 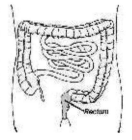 solution is retained for at least five to ten minutes to obtain the maximal effect. Find something with which to distract the bottom, like spanking his ass — yes, that'll distract him! Butt plugs come in handy for retention. If anal fisting is on the agenda, then I like to use two of the disposable enemas, because cleanliness is next to... making sure there is enough room for my whole hand!

Klismaphilia, or the use of enemas for sexual stimulation, is a practice enjoyed by a certain segment of the population, both male and female. To put it simply, klismaphilia is a type of anal play that stimulates intensive sexual feelings in some individuals. This isn't always a dominance issue; some people find that by stretching the bowel with a large enema they receive fantastic sexual stimulation. It may be due to pressure on the internal pelvic organs, which can't be provided any way from the outside. Erotic enemas aren't for everyone, but those that love them, love them a lot, judging from the amount of fan sites and equipment available. If you're going to play with enemas, play safely. Use the shut-off valve and, as with everything, if it hurts when you don't want it to, something is wrong, so stop and check it out. I refer you to the Resource Guide, which lists some outstanding references on large volume enemas, for more detailed information.

The rectum is a powerful muscular organ about five inches long, with a sphincter at each end. The sigmoid colon is a looped section of the bowel just above the rectum. It is shaped somewhat like a question mark. The loop occurs at about a depth of ten inches, as can be felt if you push a firm object into the rectum, and up through the inner sphincter. And why would we push a firm object into the rectum, through the inner sphincter? For your own good, my dear bottom, for your own good.

Now, shall we speculate on rectal dilation, a technique that requires more relaxation than stretching?

Speculums come in two flavors: vaginal and anal. Graves speculums are the most commonly used type of speculum. This vaginal speculum is shaped sort of like a duck's bill, and once it is inserted into the vaginal canal it can be gently widened to spread the interior vaginal walls. This metal speculum is sometimes used by kinksters for rectal exams as well, thrifty folks are we. Plastic, disposable vaginal speculums are

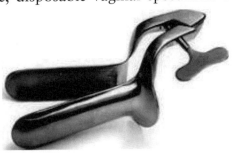

not recommended for the ass because the weak plastic may shatter and cut. Speculums are available in three sizes because vaginas are available in different sizes.

Made of strong plastic, the proctoscope is used to examine the inside of a patient's rectum. Once inserted, the inner piece with ring tab can be removed to for better visibility during the exam. When the inner tab is removed, the outer part resembles a funnel.

The large steel rectal anoscope allows you to look deep into the rectum. Once inserted, the inner shaft is removed, leaving a hollow opening. The insertable portion of the shaft is six inches long with a 3/4-inch diameter. Great for humiliating anal medical exam scenes.

Sims Stainless Steel anal scope is used to spread tissue for anal examination. The probe section is about 3.25" long, and is 3/4" in diameter when closed. When opened, the prongs spread to a maximum of 1.7" apart.

Cleaning your instruments after use is vitally important for personal safety and instrument long life. Expensive instruments have been damaged by inappropriate methods. Follow this step by step procedure for safety and success.

1. Have an established area to deposit all used instruments. This both keeps them from being reused and from contaminating other things. A plastic five gallon pail with a handle works well and allows you to carry the in-

struments to your cleaning area without dirtying yourself.

2. To protect yourself, put on a pair of exam or rubber gloves before beginning.

3. Wash everything in hot soapy water using a cloth to scrub all surfaces. This removes lubricants, fecal matter, blood, and other debris. This step is important. Sanitation and sterilization may not be able to get through surface contamination to remove germs. Both bleach and heat can cause germs to be encapsulated in a way that protects them from sanitation and sterilization. Wash rectal thermometers and other tem-

perature sensitive items in cold soapy water.

4. Rinse each item in cold water to remove soap.

5. Soak each item in a bleach solution for five minutes. The bleach solution is one cup liquid bleach to 2 quarts of water. Use a plastic container for this solution, as it will attack metal!

6. Dry each item and inspect for cracks and other damage. Discard items that should no longer be used.

Your instrument is now clean and sanitized. It is ready for storage. Think of stainless steel as stain-*less* rather than stain-*free*. Excess exposure to bleach and other strong oxidizing agents will cause it to corrode and pit, so examine your instruments before use.

Another form of moist heat that can be used to sanitize, as opposed to sterilize, is the heat-drying cycle of an automatic dishwasher. By loading pre-cleaned instruments or equipment, and not using any detergent or rinse agent, the steam from the drying cycle will effectively sanitize even interior surfaces. Run the equipment through the full wash cycle including heat drying.

One well-known BDSM company has been thinking outside the box to come up with a clever idea to delivering lube to the proper place, which is in the bottom, not all over the sheets. For less than $6 they have paired a luer-lock syringe (screw type) and a rectal tube from an enema kit. This set-up appears ideal for siphoning your favorite lube into those hard-to-reach areas. If you have access to the two parts of this "applicator," then you could make your own. To use, just screw the plastic nozzle (rectal tube) onto the syringe. Insert the end of the tube into the lube bottle. Pull back on the plunger to fill the syringe with lube. Insert into the proper orifice and push the plunger of the syringe to "inject" the lube. No muss, no fuss. Whatever you do, don't reinsert that used tube back into that bottle or you will have just contaminated the lube.

Please remember that while toys, tools and instruments can be shared with proper protection and disinfection, lube should not. A hand or syringe moving from a lube container to a person and then back to the lube container inevitably deposits things from the person to the lube container. Reserve a lube container for that bottom, or, better yet, a bottom should have his or her own lube container. My personal preference is for individual packets of lube, which, though a little more pricey, are guaranteed free from contamination.

CHAPTER 7. MEDICAL BONDAGE

Mention "medical bondage" and the first thing that pops into most people's minds is a body wrapped head to toe in bandages. Come on, you've seen "The Curse of the Mummy" too many times! Nowadays, we've got newer and more devious ways to put our bottoms into medical bondage.

While bandage wraps can still be used for a full body wrap, they can also be used as an aside to immobilize part of a person's body: lower limbs to each other, for instance; or to attach part of the body to a fixed point, such as attaching the bottom's arms to the arms of a chair.

The newest type of bandage wraps make versatile blindfolds and gags, even entire hoods at the spur of the moment. These new wraps are soft, not binding like rope, drape to fit the shape of the subject, and are easily cut with scissors. Available in a variety of colors, you can buy this self-adhesive wrap as Vet-Wrap from animal supply stores or sites or as Coban or Co-flex at pharmacies or medical supply sites. The two best features are that the new wraps are self-adhesive (that is, they stick to themselves without sticking to the bottom's skin, hair or clothing), and that they are breathable. You can wrap one or two layers over a bottom's mouth and nose, but they can still breathe through it.

The old stand-by Ace™ bandage has

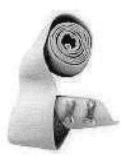

fallen by the wayside as this lighter and more breathable bandage has been filling the toybags. But Ace-type bandages still have their use, especially if you don't lose the claw attachments!

Remember this? In the final episode of season five of M*A*S*H, Hot Lips Houlihan gets married to Lt. Col. Donald Penobscot. But when Donald gets drunk at his bachelor party and passes out, Hawkeye and B.J. place him in a body cast and convince him that he has broken his leg. The ceremony is performed and Donald and Hot Lips leave for their honeymoon with him still in the fake cast. Talk about a mind-fuck!

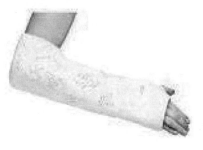

If you want to preserve a hard memory of the scene or put your patient in some serious bondage for a few hours, then break out the casting materials. Unless you have a special saw for cutting through a cast, stick with the craft-type plaster of paris impregnated gauze strips found at arts and crafts stores, such as Rigid Wrap . Alternatively, Johnson and Johnson makes plaster bandage casting supplies, available at medical supply stores. However, this product should be used with a stockinette, a soft, knitted cotton wrap, as a first layer, protecting the skin from the plaster bandages. To aid in removal of the cast, coat the area with petroleum jelly before applying the bandages. Then cut the gauze strips to a reasonable length, dip in water to activate the plastic, and lay them one by one on the area to be casted. Smooth out the strip, adding more strips to make the cast thicker. The cast may take 15 minutes of drying time. You may want to cast a breast/chest area, face (remembering to leave breathing holes), genitals, ass, or limbs. Remember to keep the cast thin enough to remove with strong scissors.

Dental gags are fiendish-looking stainless steel devices that are used by dentists and oral surgeons to keep mouths open during examinations and surgeries. If you've ever had a root canal, you may be very familiar with the Jennings Gag or Whitehead Gag with ratchet spreaders, which measure 5.5" from end to end. Bondage enthusiasts find them useful for keeping the mouth open for other reasons, i.e. humiliation, insertion of objects or body parts. Because these items were designed as medical devices, and not secure BDSM gags, it is generally possible to push them out of the mouth with some effort.

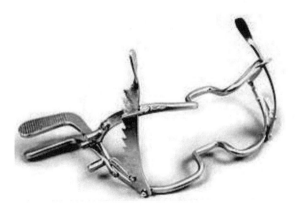

However, adding some sort of strap around the back of the head will make them more secure. Consider wrapping parts of the gag in tape to prevent chipping teeth against the hard metal. Also take care not to strain the jaw muscles by opening the jaw too much or for too long.

The "H" shaped, spring-loaded dental gag is a more evil gag that keeps the bottom's mouth wide open — but unlike the Jennings or Whitehead gags, the bottom won't be able to push it out. Here is how it works: squeeze it so that it is only about an inch in length. Insert it into the bottom's mouth. As he or she opens their mouth to speak, the dental gag will automatically widen up to three inches. The gag cannot be pushed out of the mouth due to the two plastic stoppers set behind the teeth. To remove, use your fingers to press the rear of the gag to allow it to close again. Why am I getting flashbacks of the dental office scene from "Little Shop of Horrors?"

Finally, nobody knows medical bondage better than the psychiatric hospital caretakers, right, Nurse Ratched? Go rent a copy of *One Flew Over the Cuckoo's Nest* to see a plethora of institutional restraints put to use. Canvas restraining wraps make people-enchiladas by basically wrapping a person in a small canvas blanket that has Velcro or buckling fasteners and handles for carrying. Arm and leg restraints work the same way: wrap tightly around the limb, fasten with super-strong Velcro, then the other end can be used to attach the bottom to a fixed point, as a leash, or brought around the body to immobilize that limb. Don't mistake these institutional restraints for the flimsy Velcro beginner's bondage sets sold in adult stores. Psychiatric restraints were designed to be strong and escape-proof.

Of course the ultimate in institutional restraint is the handy-dandy straitjacket. Traditionally, it's a reasonably tough fabric garment designed to prevent violent mentally disturbed patients and prisoners from causing harm to themselves and

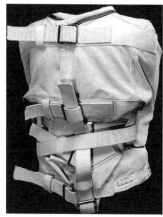

other people before the days of sedatives. Straitjackets or strait-waistcoats can be anything from a simple smock with closed sleeve ends and tie tapes, to deliberately intimidating constructions of canvas, leather straps and metal hardware. These are designed to help safely control the most aggressive patient. Long-sleeved arms cross in front of the bottom before buckling in back. The pelvic strap effectively prevents the bottom from pulling the jacket over the head.

CHAPTER 8. URETHRAL PLAY: SOUNDS LIKE FUN

Urethral play is the red-headed stepchild of the BDSM world, misunderstood or overlooked. My mission the past few years has been to deflower as many urethras as possible and educate my community to the pleasures of UP, particularly tops who have female bottoms. It's time to wake up and grab those urethral sounds and catheters, because you are missing out on some heavy-duty orgasms.

To insert or have something inserted into the urethra can be a very pleasurable experience, for both men and women. The urethra is a very sensitive organ and stretching it slightly can provide some exquisite sexual pleasure. If sounds are used correctly, with plenty of lubrication and without exceeding the appropriate size for the bottom, there should be no real pain. There may be some initial discomfort, which will give way to great pleasure after the first anxious moments. You must start with the smaller ones and work up to the larger sizes. It will dilate the urethra somewhat for a short period of time, but will return to normal, just like in ass play.

It's hard to explain what it feels like. There's a combination of stretching, awkwardness, invasion, comfort, pain, pleasure and all the psychological aspects of being violated in such a way.

It is difficult to compare this sensation to anything you've ever experienced, although my male partner describes it as a hand-job from the inside or as a long, slow orgasm. For women, the urethra is located directly above the vagina, so it is similarly innervated. Many women find that when their urethra is probed, it feels like being fucked.

Men's urinary tracts are a bit complicated, not as simple as women's. The reason is that the urethra in men has two functions, transporting urine and the semen. Another complicating factor is the matter of erections: one minute the penis is flaccid and only a couple inches long, next minute it can be erect and several inches long. The full length of the male urethra ranges from 11.5 to 13 inches. Also the urethra in itself is not used to having an intruder push in and is rather sticky. For these reasons, sounds used by men are very different, and much more particular about their shape, than sounds or dilators used by women.

Sounds are constructed of stainless surgical steel or chrome-plated brass and normally are purchased from a medical supply store. They are probably the best option for long term usage and come in many different shapes and sizes. The Pratt sounds are to be considered the "male sounds" and are straight for the most part, with the exception of the ends that are bent at a 10-15 degree angle. The Hegar are considered the "female sounds" and are curved in a slight "S" shape.

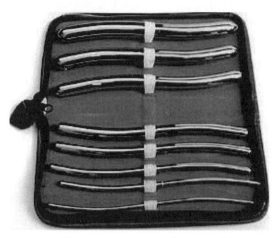

(Actually Hegar sounds are dilators and are used to dilate the cervix, but work beautifully with the urethra.) Sounds usually come in sets containing 8 or 9 each, ranging from a tiny 2mm to a whopping 18mm. Whichever size suits you, these Hegar are perfect for the beginner: they can be inserted in an erect cock because they have only a gentle curve but are not long enough to reach the prostate, and because they're not too long, are perfect for the female urethra as well.

There are also Van Buren sounds, which are much thinner and curved, and Dittel sounds, which are rather like Van Buren's without the bend in the end. Van Buren sounds are for going all the way to the bladder and should not be inserted in an erect cock. Bakes, also called "rosebud" sounds because of a little bud or bullet at the end of a thin straight rod, can massage the prostate.

Even if you are not into urethral play, you never know when you are going to have to put a bottom into strict bondage for an extended length of time that may interfere with accessibility to the bathroom. Unless you have them

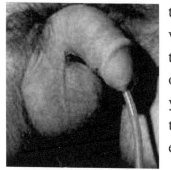 tied up out in the woods and intend to let them piss on themselves, you may want to consider catheterization.

But if the idea of inserting a catheter is too scary or invasive for you, or your bottom is backed into a corner yelling, "RED, RED, RED," don't despair of never having an extended session with your bondage boy. I've got just what the doctor ordered: external catheters, also known as condom catheters or Texas catheters for males. Don't forget the leg bags and tubing and you have everything needed for a no-excuses all-nighter with your male bottom.

External catheters fit like a condom and come in small, intermediate and "in your dreams." Remember that this is sized upon a flaccid state. Because the catheters are already treated with an adhesive, just roll one down the cock and it stays there until you take it off. External catheters are available at home health stores, medical supply stores and many pharmacies.

Urethral play is invasive, potentially risky, takes practice, and should be learned from someone who knows what they are doing — an experienced SM player and/or medical professional. Proper sanitary procedure is essential — you don't want to give your bottom a bladder or genital infection. There are Yahoo groups devoted to this fetish, many articles on the web to guide you, and kinky companies who will instruct you as they sell their products to you. Do your homework, respect the risks, and have fun!

Chapter 9. Scalpel, Please — Breaking Skin

"**B**loodsports" is a generic name for any SM practice that involves blood. Properly done, none of these practices result in any damage that requires more than minor first aid to clean up and cope with. However, a mistake could lead to serious and permanent injury. You need to learn from an experienced top, and you need to see it done in person, before playing this way with your partners.

In any medical scene with piercing of the skin, your approach to sterility should mirror that of an actual doctor.

Sterility is essential, from the supplies you buy to the play areas in your "office." When you buy your piercing needles, some medical supply houses offer ethylene oxide gas sterilization. Ethylene oxide gas sterilization is an effective way — equivalent to autoclaving — to sterilize most medical play items. Anything used to break skin, unless it's fresh out of a sterile package, should be sterilized using this method. Once sterilized in this way, the items are sealed in plastic and are germ free until you use them. (Use disposable needles once and throw them away as medical waste.)

Before you start your session, wash your hands thoroughly with a hospital quality anti-bacterial soap. Disposable exam gloves should be placed on both hands immediately after washing. The bottom's skin should also be cleaned with an anti-bacterial wash to kill any residual skin bacteria. You should have all these products on hand, neatly arranged on your medical table, so that the doctor role-play and the sterility precautions you are taking merge seamlessly. Here is a great area where real life and role-play completely intersect. Bottoms: As in any doctor/patient relationship, the "patient" should make sure that the "doctor" is as professional as possible — or leave the office!

Play piercings are a relatively mild form of bloodsports. The needles used are sterile hypodermic needles available from medical supply stores or serious SM shops. The top pinches up a bit of skin and slides the needle through. Each needle doesn't necessarily hurt that much, but your nerves definitely know it's there, and the endorphins start to flow very quickly. After a while, the needles are removed and put into a disposable sharps container, and the bottom gets Band-Aids™ if any are needed, although generally the holes are small enough that they clot immediately.

Cutting is the SM practice of using a scalpel or other fine blade to make shallow cuts in the top layer of your partner's skin, at about the depth of a cat scratch. The usual instrument for cutting is a surgical scalpel, which is sharp enough to make a smooth, clean cut; using duller blades can leave a ragged cut that doesn't heal as well.

Cuts are made on areas of the body where the skin is not stretched tight: for example, the shoulder blade, or the buttock, or the front of the thigh. Cuts are not made anywhere that the skin becomes taut, since such places won't heal well because the cut will keep getting pulled open. Only one layer of skin is cut — the very topmost layer. Deeper cuts don't heal well. And cuttings generally don't form loops, as the skin in the center of the loop can be cut off from its blood supply. When the cutting is complete, the whole area is generally bandaged. The best safety advice: be taught by someone who knows how to do cuttings safely.

Suturing, stapling, cauterizing, infusion, injection and scarification are all extreme medical play that go beyond the scope of this little manual. Anyone wanting to explore those areas should do their homework thoroughly, train under the tutelage of an experienced top or medical practitioner, have the proper tools and use the utmost care. I encourage you to delve into these areas as they the "cutting edge" of medical

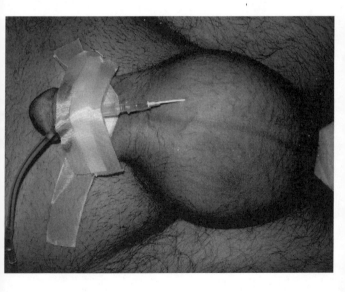

play and the most exciting! Don't you think that my husband's scrotum looks very excited to be infused with a liter of saline?

REFERENCES AND RESOURCES

Addington, Deborah. *Play Piercing*. Oakland, CA, Greenery Press, 2006.

Body Modification E-zine: www.bmezine.com

Bush G, Nixon RK. Scrotal inflation: A new cause for subcutaneous, mediastinal and retroperitoneal emphysema. Henry Ford Hosp Med J 1969; 17: 225-226.

Chase Union web site: www.chaseunion.com

CMHurt: www.cmhurt.com

Enema Lover's Guide: www.enemaloversguide.com

Extreme Restraints: www.extremer-estraints.com

Fozzie's Den: www.fozden.com

Frau Doktor: www.fraudoktor.com/medical/eindex.htm

Fun Products: www.funproducts.com/index.html

Healthy and Active: www.healthyan-dactive.com/index.html

Hussain NA, Warshaw G. Utility of clysis for hydration in nursing home residents. J Am Geriatr Soc 1996; 44: 969-973.

Strict, M.R. *Intimate Invasions: The Erotic Ins and Outs of Enema Play.* Oakland, CA, Greenery Press, 2004.

JT's Stockroom: www.stockroom.com

Kinky Medical: www.kinkymedical.net

Kittens Toy Room: www.kittenstoyroom.com/

Leatherpost: www.leatherpost.com

Love B. *The Encyclopedia of Unusual Sex Practices.* Fort Lee, NJ, Barricade Books, 1992.

medical Toys: www.medicaltoys.com/

Rainbow Rope: www.rainbowrope.com

Rupert Huse & Son: www.huse.com

Sharma TC, Kagan HN. Scrotal emphysema. Am Surg 1980; 46: 652-653.

Surgical911: www.surgical911.com/index.html

Whirlwind Distributing: www.brownbottle.com

www.bmezine.com/extreme/free/cmhurt/saline.html

www.harmful.org/homedespot/newtdr/newtdrarchive/gothic/medicalparty.htm

TOYBAG GUIDES: A Workshop In A Book   *$9.95 each*

Canes and Caning, by Janet Hardy

Clips and Clamps, by Jack Rinella

Erotic Knifeplay, by Miranda Austin and Sam Atwood

Foot and Shoe Worship, by Midori

Hot Wax and Temperature Play, by Spectrum

Dungeon Emergencies & Supplies, by Jay Wiseman

BDSM/KINK

The Compleat Spanker
Lady Green $12.95

Erotic Tickling
Michael Moran $13.95

Family Jewels: A Guide to Male Genital Play and Torment
Hardy Haberman $12.95

Flogging
Joseph W. Bean $12.95

Intimate Invasions: The Ins and Outs of Erotic Enema Play
M.R. Strict $13.95

Jay Wiseman's Erotic Bondage Handbook
Jay Wiseman $16.95

The Kinky Girl's Guide to Dating
Luna Grey $16.95

The Loving Dominant
John Warren $16.95

Miss Abernathy's Concise Slave Training Manual
Christina Abernathy $12.95

The Mistress Manual: The Good Girl's Guide to Female Dominance
Mistress Lorelei $16.95

Play Piercing
Deborah Addington $13.95

Radical Ecstasy: SM Journeys to Transcendence
Dossie Easton and Janet W. Hardy $16.95

The Sexually Dominant Woman: A Workbook for Nervous Beginners
Lady Green $11.95

The Seductive Art of Japanese Bondage
Midori $27.95

Please include $3 for first book and $1 for each additional book with your order to cover shipping and handling costs, plus $10 for overseas orders.

GREENERY PRESS

SM 101: A Realistic Introduction
Jay Wiseman $24.95

GENERAL SEXUALITY

Big Big Love: A Sourcebook on Sex for People of Size and Those Who Love Them
Hanne Blank $15.95

The Bride Wore Black Leather... And He Looked Fabulous!: An Etiquette Guide for the Rest of Us
Andrew Campbell $11.95

... But I Know What You Want: 25 Sex Tales for the Different
James Williams $13.95

The Ethical Slut: A Guide to Infinite Sexual Possibilities
Dossie Easton & Catherine A. Liszt $16.95

Fantasy Made Flesh: The Essential Guide to Erotic Roleplay
Deborah Addington $13.95

A Hand in the Bush: The Fine Art of Vaginal Fisting
Deborah Addington $13.95

Health Care Without Shame: A Handbook for the Sexually Diverse and Their Caregivers
Charles Moser, Ph.D., M.D. $11.95

Look Into My Eyes: How to Use Hypnosis to Bring Out the Best in Your Sex Life
Peter Masters $16.95

Paying For It: A Guide By Sex Workers for Their Clients
edited by Greta Christina $13.95

Phone Sex: Oral Thrills and Aural Skills
Miranda Austin $15.95

Photography for Perverts
Charles Gatewood $27.95

Sex Disasters... And How to Survive Them
Charles Moser, Ph.D., M.D. and Janet W. Hardy $16.95

Tricks... To Please a Man *and* Tricks... To Please a Woman
both by Jay Wiseman $14.95 ea.

When Someone You Love Is Kinky
Dossie Easton & Catherine A. Liszt $15.95

VISA/MC accepted. Order from Greenery Press, 4200 Park Blvd. pmb 240, Oakland, CA 94602, 510/530-1281. www.greenerypress.com.